Skincare Manual

Discover Natural Remedies and Plans to Achieve a Flawless Skin

Written by

Zaina Medina

Copyright © by Zaina Medina 2023. All Rights Reserved.

Table of Contents

Introduction

There is more to achieving healthy, glowing skin than using a ton of products or a complicated regimen. It's important to separate the essentials from the overwhelming amount of skincare advice in a world where the advice is abundant. Simplifying skincare is essential since quality always wins out over quantity.

This book eliminates the unnecessary and concentrates on essential procedures, covering everything from the need for a simplified routine such as the benefits of a brief method to attain radiant skin to specific approaches, including double cleansing for efficient makeup removal.

Professional opinions highlight the importance of skincare consistency and stress that sticking to a regimen is essential for seeing true, long-lasting benefits. Furthermore, nourishing the health of the skin requires a grasp of the complex balance of products, the order in which they should be applied, and the significance of avoiding irritants like scents and chemicals that can cause damage to your skin over time.

This book also supports preventive care, and a roadmap toward long-term skin health and brightness, not an instant transformation guarantee. Its evidence supporting the idea that the most satisfying results come from updated regular, and conscientious care, one that guarantees the vitality of your skin for ages to come.

Understanding Your Skin Type

It's critical to recognize your skin type for the purpose of maintaining it. There are the following kinds of skin:

1. Sensitive skin

Sensitive skin is the phrase used to describe skin that is readily irritated and prone to heightened reaction. This sensitive skin type can be defined by irritation, redness, itching, and increased heat sensitivity. Additionally, its barrier function is disrupted, making it easier for pathogens and germs to get inside and possibly triggering infections and allergic symptoms.

It's critical to know the difference between skin sensitivity and allergies. Allergies can cause severe symptoms, which can include nausea and difficulty breathing. However, skin sensitivity is not always implied by allergies, such as dust allergies. You may not have sensitive skin generally, but you may be allergic to a particular chemical in skincare products.

Conversely, strong chemicals and some skincare products can cause responses in those with sensitive skin.

Sensitive skin requires careful attention to detail. Patch tests must be performed before to employing new products in order to prevent negative responses. It is advised to streamline the skincare regimen by using gentle cleansers, moisturizers, and sunscreen.

Choose lotions and cleansers without sulfates that have calming ingredients like chamomile or green tea. Contrary to common assumption, items with the label "hypoallergenic" may not be suited for everyone and require patch testing before to use. Additionally, by retaining vital oils on sensitive skin, avoiding long, hot showers helps stop additional discomfort.

Use a gentle facial cleanser to wash your face, then rinse with warm water. Gently dry your skin softly rather than rubbing it with a cloth. Sensitive skin may get irritated by exfoliation. Avoid using products that contain scent, soap, alcohol, or acid. Instead, seek for nutrients like oats, green tea polyphenols, chamomile, and aloe on the label that are known to be calming. Your face might look happier if a product has fewer components.

2. Normal skin

Normal skin is clear, balanced, and insensitive skin. When washing your face, don't just use whatever soap is available at the sink or in the shower. Additionally, don't feel pressured to purchase ostentatious or costly items. Simply choose a skin care regimen that suits you.

Using your fingertips, gently apply soap or a light cleaner on the normal skin. Avoid washing your face. After rinsing with lots of warm water, pat dry.

Try using a different cleanser if your skin becomes greasy or dries up.

3. Dry skin

The skin type that generates less sebum than typical is referred to as "Dry Skin." The skin that's dry lacks the lipids required to hold onto moisture and provide a barrier against outside effects because it produces insufficient sebum. Dry skin can be rough, scaly, or crumbly.

Use a mild cleanser without alcohol or scents for this type of skin. You may become even more dehydrated from those components.

After giving your skin a gentle wash, thoroughly rinse with warm water. Avoid using hot water on your face as it will quickly eliminate the body's own low level moisturizers.

Once a week exfoliation can help remove dry skin cells. Your skin will appear more even and brighter as a result.

4. Oily skin

An oily skin type is one that produces more sebum than normal. We refer to this surplus production as seborrhea. This kind of skin could have large pores and is oily and glossy.

Wash your face using a foamy cleanser that is free of oil. Use lots of warm water to rinse. After, you could wish to use an astringent or toner, but proceed with caution since it could irritate your skin. The aforementioned items can help maintain clean skin and eliminate excess oil, which lessens the shine on your face.

5. Mixed Skin

As the name implies, mixed or combination skin is skin that has elements of several different skin types - both oily and dry skin. This kind of skin has oily areas on the forehead, nostrils, and chin. Since it is oilier than the rest of the skin and more vulnerable to ultraviolet (UV) rays, it needs to be adequately shielded from sunlight.

A customized skincare regimen is essential for people navigating the challenging terrain of mixed skin. With its increased pores, the T-zone (area constituting the forehead, nostril and chin) frequently presents a special difficulty that requires careful attention.

First, cleansing turns into a careful balance; it's important to use gentle cleanser that remove pollutants from the skin without clogging pores.

Although useful, exfoliation needs to be done at a controlled pace. Excessive exfoliating may remove vital oils from the skin, leaving it vulnerable. Therefore, it is recommended to follow a mild and infrequent exfoliation regimen, avoiding harsh scrubbing in the T-zone area to avoid unintentional skin injury.

Protecting oneself from the sun's powerful illuminates is a must. For people with combination skin, selecting an oil-free sunscreen acts as a barrier against potential skin issues.

Recognizing that products designed for dry skin might not be compatible with the requirements of oily areas, it is wise to keep distinct routines for the T-zone and other areas of the face. Different moisturizers address different needs: rich density for the cheekbones and a lighter, oil-free alternative for the erratic T-zone.

Furthermore, those products themselves are included in the list of skincare allies.

Choosing oil-free formulas for everything cosmetics and sunscreen included lowers the chance of pore obstruction. The selection of natural products free of fragrances that provide comfort to combination skin that is prone to flare-ups is equally important. For individuals looking for the elusive balance of combination skin care, a keen eye towards fragrance and oil-free products serves as a guiding light in the maze of skincare options.

Herbal Approaches to Natural Skin Protection

The effectiveness of herbal remedies for promoting and preserving the health of your skin is examined in this section.

- **Green Tea**

Green tea has antioxidants that can help lower toxicity and delay the aging process. For those with oily or acne-prone skin, green tea can help control sebum production thanks to these components. Their astringent qualities might aid in pore reduction and smooth the look of the skin.

- **Cucumber**

Cucumber is excellent for whitening the complexion and is also one of the simplest methods for getting rid of wrinkles, pimples, acne, and other imperfections.

Apply the juice of cucumber on your face, After 20 - 25 minutes, wash your skin, It makes your skin, eyes, and face more beautiful by getting rid of spots.

- **Tomatoes**

One of the best at-home remedies for skin care issues is the tomato. It aids skin fairness. Red tomato juice can be applied on the face.

Cut up a red tomato and apply it to your face. Rinse your face with water when it dries. If done consistently, it will assist to reduce facial wrinkles and make the skin shine.

- **Berries**

Nutrient-dense berries like blueberries and strawberries are a delightful snack. They also support the preservation of youthful skin by battling free radicals and pollutants in our skin.

- **Flaxseeds and Walnuts**

Flaxseeds and walnuts are rich in Omega 3 fatty acids, which support the treatment of skin inflammation and dry patches of skin in addition to supporting brain function.

- **Fuller's Earth**

To make a fine paste, incorporate it with rose water. On a clean face, apply. After it has totally dried off, rinse it off.

It is suggested because of its superior oil-absorbing qualities and its cooling qualities, which have a soothing impact on irritated or inflamed skin.

- **Rice Water**

To make rice water, soak some raw rice in purified water. After 30 -35 minutes of soaking, gather this water in a spray bottle. Spritz your face with this water. After 15 minutes, remove with cold water and rinse.

For skin conditions like eczema or sunburn, it is appropriate since it includes components that have the potential to relieve and calm irritation or sensitive skin. Rice water, which is high in antioxidants and minerals, may even out skin tone, brighten complexion, and lessen the visibility of pigmentation or dark spots.

- **Gram flour**

Gram flour is a great natural face cleanser for skin that is bright, whitening, acne-free, and effectively removes facial hair. Add a small amount of salt to the gram flour, knead the mixture, and apply it on your face. This will result in a vivid and lovely face.

- **Orange peel powder**

Combine the powder with curd or rosewater. After 20 minutes, wash your face with cold water to remove the product.

Because of the vitamin C it contains, it might help lighten dark spots, promote more even skin tone, and brighten the complexion. It has inherent antibacterial qualities that might aid in battling bacteria that cause acne and lessening outbreaks.

- **Lemon with Curd**

You can achieve amazing results by gently massaging your face with a spoonful of curd and a dash of lemon.

Curd's inherent moisturizing qualities can help moisturize the skin, making it feel supple and smoother. Lemon's citric acid and curd's lactic acid can both brighten skin by fading dark spots and encouraging an even more radiant appearance. While the lactic acid found in curd helps to remove dead skin cells and leave the skin smoother, lemon's natural acids gently exfoliate the skin.

- **Haldi or Tumeric and Besan**

Instead of using all of your pricey facial washes, try this. Apply a besan and haldi mixture to your face along with some milk or curd. Turmeric powder or Haldi is a medication due to its antibacterial qualities. An excellent and all-natural exfoliating ingredient is besan or chickpea flour. Apply it all over your body, if at all possible, and scrub it off once it has become somewhat dried and little untidy, but your skin will be lovely and supple afterward.

- **Aloe Vera gel**

Use aloe vera gel and rosewater on your skin after washing it before bed, and let it sit there all night. The outcomes will be visible to you in a week.

- **Sweet Potatoes and Carrots**

Sweet potatoes and carrots are high in beta carotene, which improves skin tone and eye health. Regular consumption of these will eventually result in glowing skin.

Seasonal Skin Protection

Skin is impacted by seasonal changes; for the best protection, adjust skincare to weather-related concerns like dryness, exposure to the sun, and humidity.

The following practices are recommended for seasonal changes:

❖ **Summer Season**

Every day, apply sunscreen. Use SPF sunscreen daily, regardless of your skin type or how your body responds to the sun. About shot glass of sunscreen should be reapplied at least three times a day for every part of your body. Many are unaware that even on heavily cloudy days, in cooler environments, and when they are not in sunlight for prolonged periods, they can still suffer burn.

Apart from having broad-brimmed hats and a pair of sunglasses an increasing amount of studies indicates that regular clothing items like tightly made shirts or shorts provide superior protection from the sun. Furthermore, there is high-Sun Protection Factor apparel, which is made of colorless chemicals, and specially treated polymers which absorb ultraviolet (UV) rays.

If your skin has undergone a significant alteration, avoid going outside in the sun. Early symptoms of skin cancer include hard red patches, shifting moles, and discolored skin. You ought to consult a dermatologic surgeon, who is specially trained to identify and treat skin cancer, if you observe any of these symptoms.

❖ The Winter Season

More than headgear, protective gloves, and coats are needed to protect skin from the cold in order to maintain health. Insufficient moisture from the wind and colder temperatures can lead to splitting, dryness, irritation, and skin disorders like eczema. Above all, it is imperative to maintain vigilance regarding sun safety during the winter months.

In order to assist seal in and refresh the skin with the essential water and oils, it is ideal to apply moisturizer right away after taking a bath or shower as it helps shield the skin from the damaging effects of the weather. Although taking a lengthy, hot shower is enjoyable for everyone, the hot water can deplete the skin of its natural oils, which can lead to dry skin. Use warm water instead, but for a shorter duration.

Putting on gloves is a quick and easy method to shield your hands from the dry air and cold that can cause dermatitis. Don't forget to use sunscreen because the sun's UV rays are still very strong in the winter because snow reflects sunlight. If you engage in winter sports without wearing sunscreen, you run the risk of getting very badly burned.

Both men and women should use lip moisturizer or lipsticks with a high sun protection factor throughout the winter.

❖ Fall Season

The arrival of dry, colder air can cause skin to lose vital hydration. It also offers a chance to repair the damage that sun, chlorine, and seawater caused to skin during the summer. To assist with seal in and restore the skin with the essential water and oils, it's recommended to use moisturizer right after a bath or shower. Skin requires a heavier moisturizer when the air gets drier.

Maintain your defenses against the sun's radiation. In order to avoid having dry, lips that are cracked, start moisturizing now as well. Creams offer a more robust greasy barrier to keep moisture in. Wintertime often causes hands to become dry and cracked. In order to maintain soft and healthier hands throughout, start hydrating them now. Despite the seemingly lower temperatures and shorter days, both adults and children should still apply sunscreen before venturing outside.

❖ Spring Season

Even if it's getting warmer outside and people can spend more time outside , there are still some crucial things to be aware of that may help prevent skin damage from the sun. The SPF of a sunscreen lotion should vary according to the skin's pigmentation, which might affect the chance of burning in the sun. For instance, your skin is more vulnerable to UV radiation if you have freckles and are fair-skinned.

Every year, have your skin screened by a dermatological surgeon to find out what precautions you should take.

Creating a Personalized Skincare Plan

Create a personalized skincare regimen for radiant, healthy skin by selecting products and techniques that suits your needs.

The following are healthy and comprehensive skin care plans for sunrise and dawn;

Sunrise

1. Use a low-pH cleaner to cleanse

Utilize a product with a low pH cleanser, like CeraVe Hydrating Cleanser or COSRX Low-pH Good Morning Cleanser 150ml.

2. Use hyaluronic acid serum to add elasticity and moisture

Products like Purito Pure Hyaluronic Acid 90 Serum and Luisa Fanzani Hyaluronic Acid absorb water, perk up the skin, and increase elasticity.

3. Include Vitamin C Serum for radiance and defense

Vitamin C serum, such as Louisa Fanzani's 10% or The Ordinary's 23%, is a beneficial antioxidant that improves skin and reduces fine wrinkles.

4. Sooth yourself with a moisturizing cream

Apply a calming moisture lotion like I'm From Mugwort lotion or Dear, Klairs Rich Moist Soothing Cream.

Skincare Manual

5. Sun Defense

Use a sunscreen that protects your skin, such as Beauty of Joseon Relief Sun, Rice + Probiotics or Garnier Ombrelle Ultra Light Advanced Face Lotion SPF 50+.

For an undetectable tint and sun protection, use BB Creams like Dr. Jart Silver Label BB Cream or Klairs Illuminating Supple Blemish Cream SPF40.

Dawn

1. Start with using Bioderma H20 Micellar Water on an absorbent cotton (pay attention to your skin type) get rid of sunscreen and facial makeup.

2. For the second cleaning, use a low-pH foamy cleanser like CeraVe Salicylic Acid

Cleanser or COSRX low-pH Good Morning Cleanser.

3. Use a liquid exfoliator, like Paula's Choice, 2% BHA Liquid, also known as ordinary glycolic acid 7% Toning Solution. Liquid exfoliates are essential for removing debris from pores, minimizing wrinkles, and balancing the tone of the skin.

4. Use a retinoid, the most common ingredient in anti-aging products, such as Paula's Choice 1% Retinol Treatment or The Ordinary Retinol 0.5% in Squalane, to promote collagen, eliminate wrinkles, remove pigmentation, and prevent acne on days when you don't use a liquid exfoliation.

5. **Hydration**: To hydrate, repair, and recover skin after exfoliation, apply a high proportion of snail mucus or propolis serum (such as Cosrx Advanced Snail Mucin Power Essence or Propolis B5 Glow Barrier Calming Serum).

6. Vitamin B3, diminishes pore size, congestion, uneven skin tone, and lightens the appearance of post-blemish marks like Paula's Choice. 10% or 20% serum niacinamide

7. **Moisturize**: Apply a calming moisture lotion like I'm From Mugwort lotion or Klairs Rich Moist Soothing Cream.

Tips for Effective Skincare

It's crucial to heed your doctor's advice and remember the following pointers in order to safeguard your skin.

Nutritional Tips

1. Lemon water (warm)

I consume a glass of lemon water that is warm upon an empty stomach first thing each day when I wake up. It gives me flawless skin by assisting me in eliminating all of the toxins that are present in my body.

2. Eat a Balanced Diet

Eat a healthy, well-balanced diet. Consume a lot of fruits, whole grains, lean meats, and other nutrients to provide your skin with the nutrients it needs to be healthy and consume a lot of vegetables, proteins (meat and seafood contain collagen), omega 3 fatty acids (found in salmon, avocado, etc.), and antioxidants (found in berries, green tea, and turmeric). Wheatgrass juice and beansprouts are also excellent for reviving skin and enhancing its radiance.

3. Stay Hydrated

Maintaining hydration for your skin is a recommendation that most dermatologists would undoubtedly agree with. Water is necessary for all body processes to proceed without interruption.

Your body can experience dry, flaky skin and a host of other skin issues when it fails to receive enough water from the inside. Every day, consume between eight and ten glasses of water. Dermatologists advise that getting adequate water into your body would help with most skin issues. Water is an excellent way to remove toxins off the skin and body, so make sure you drink plenty of it!

Lifestyle Tips

It is essential to cleanse the skin before bed in order to get rid of dust, pollutants, and expired makeup.

1. Examine ingredients on skin care products with caution

Understanding the contents on the labels of the skin care products you use may either benefit or damage your skin. Steer clear of comedogenic products, alcohol, perfumes, sulfates, and preservatives. Choose glycerin-containing products that provide hydrating elements for dry skin. Your skin is safer when the items are softer. Depending on your particular preferences, you might also wish to take into account natural, organic, and vegan products. Rather of being unduly harsh on your skin, use moderate skincare products. Excessive usage of products ages the skin.

To achieve healthy, radiant skin, always choose for natural products instead of chemical-based ones.

2. **Apply a generous amount of sunscreen**

Sunlight's damaging rays are the number one cause of skin damage. Although the sun provides a good source of vitamin D, avoid receiving too much of it on your face. Severe sun exposure accelerates the aging process and causes age spots, hyperpigmentation, and other skin conditions. The only thing saving you is a high-quality sunscreen.

3. Use Face wash

Instead of soap, use a face wash or gentle cleansers because those beauty bars with their high pH might harm your skin. Dried-out, irritated skin, allergic responses, and other problems can be brought on by harsh soaps. It is advisable to change to face washes with a pH that is gentler on your skin and moderate cleansers. The optimal pH is 7, but soaps typically have a pH of 9 or 10, which might destroy all the extra care you are providing for your skin.

4. Work out frequently

More blood is pumped by the heart to the cells when you do this, which produces more oxygen.

This procedure aids in the turnover of cells. Sweating also unclogs pores, but make sure to constantly remove sweat afterward.

5. Use a fresh towel on your face

You may be surprised to learn that using the same towels over and over again might lead to the spread of bacteria and skin irritations. Never lend out your towel to someone else. The key to clear skin is to keep things tidy.

6. Antioxidants

Whether you apply them topically or consume them internally, antioxidants are really good for your skin. Try to incorporate them into your routine. Antioxidants mitigate the deleterious impact of free radicals on skin cells. Free radicals can exacerbate UV damage, therefore it's important to take your regular dose of antioxidants.

7. Sleep

When you sleep, your entire body and skin cells heal themselves. Don't deny your skin the advantages that come from getting enough sleep. Dermatologists advise getting 7- 8 hours of sleep each day.

8. Be constant

Above all else in importance. You won't see the best effects if you don't take continuous care of your skin. It's not what anyone wants to hear. People would rather hear that they can look ten years younger in an instant by simply applying serum a few times which won't make you see achieve the flawless skin.

Things Not To Do

Use no more than necessary products: Applying several skincare products at once should be avoided. It may be too abrasive for the skin, causing irritation and additional outbreaks.

1. Reduce your intake of junk food

Although it may be boring to you with this, dermatologists claim that reducing your intake of harmful junk food would greatly improve your skin. While some cheat days are acceptable a balanced, healthy diet will have a remarkable impact on your skin.

2. Don't Smoke

Smoking damages the fibers called collagen and elastin, which give your skin its strength and suppleness. Drinking too much and smoking can harm your skin and accelerate the aging process.

3. Excessive sugar

Sugar can also cause the skin to lose its suppleness and age prematurely.

4. Stress

Learn to manage your stress in a variety of situations. Unmanaged stress can make your skin more sensitive, trigger breakouts of acne, and result in other skin problems. Discover good coping mechanisms for your stress, including yoga, meditation, or exercise, as prolonged stress can cause inflammation and breakouts.

5. Coffee-based beverages

These can cause your body to become dehydrated, which can result in scaly, itchy, and dry skin.

6. Avoid compressing pimples

This can cause the bacteria and infection to get more deeply embedded, causing inflammation and extending the duration of hyperpigmentation.

Conclusion

It's critical to have a dermatologist examine your entire body and to check your moles on a regular basis, at least once a year. Particularly if you enjoy spending time in the sun or reside in a country with a warm environment.

After waking up, have one or two glasses of warm water with a fresh lemon. This ought to detoxify your system and control your bowel movements. You may tell how well you are taking care of yourself by looking at your urine and bowel motion. Maintaining your internal fitness is crucial. Make an effort to replace the sugar you consume with fruits. Make sure you eat salad on a regular basis. For excellent skin, the more vibrant your pallet, the better. Be sure to stay hydrated.

And don't forget to sleep! Nothing but a lack of sleep will be a more telling sign of fatigue on our faces.

It's crucial to keep in mind that using a natural skin care product on a regular basis will maximize its benefits. When utilizing artificial components in skincare products, some frequent errors people make are; using them excessively or not taking them at the suggested times.

To My Respected Audience

We appreciate your suggestions very greatly! Please take a moment to provide a review after reading my work. Your suggestion helps me develop as a writer. I'm grateful.

www.ingramcontent.com/pod-product-compliance
Lightning Source LLC
Chambersburg PA
CBHW070738260726